Impact of Communication in the Healthcare Field:

A Guide for Healthcare Professionals

I0475440

Author: Carol Taylor

EJD Health Law, MS Human Resource Management,

& MS in Marriage and Family Therapy

About The Author,

Carol Taylor is the founder of Solution Focused Consulting Group and brings a vast amount of knowledge from various disciplines. Below is a listing of Carol's educational Vitae.

1. Bachelor's Degree in Mathematics Education
2. Master's Degree in Marriage and Family Therapy
3. Master's Degree in Human Resource Management
4. EJD with emphasis in Health Law

The combination of these degrees creates a field of knowledge that is comprehensive and in doing so, allows Carol to approach many work environment problems from many angles; such as, employee relationships, effective communication and legalities surrounding a number of business models.

Experience:

Carol Taylor has experience working in a Human Resource department within a medical setting. This involved creating job descriptions, an employee handbook and a compensation plan based on the company's goals. These responsibilities also included creating performance plans and evaluations in order to increase deficiencies in low customer service ratings within a dental organization.

She has spent ten years working as a trainer and re-trainer within an educational and business environment. In addition, she designed a training manual for teaching new employees how to build rapport with potential customers, display empathy, and how to be productive within a business environment. With her Human Resource experience and counseling background, Carol Taylor is effective in building long-term relationships with customers, which is imperative in a business environment.

In addition, she has several years of educational experience in teaching Medical Law and Ethics to students who are being trained in health professional careers.

Acknowledgements

The author would like to thank the physicians, dentists and staff who participated in the survey, which assisted in the research findings. I would like to give a special thanks to Dr. Élan Salee for arranging the personal interviews, sending the surveys to the health care professionals, and helping me modify the physician and dentist rating scale. Additionally, I would like to thank my husband, Leith Taylor (MFT & MCTE), for his understanding and assistance throughout the editing process. In addition, I would like to thank Tonya Hundley for her hours of reading and re-editing. Last but not least, I would like to recognize Dr. Barrett for his assistance and guidance while helping me through the review of the materials as it was compiled.

TABLE OF CONTENTS

Chapter 1

Introduction

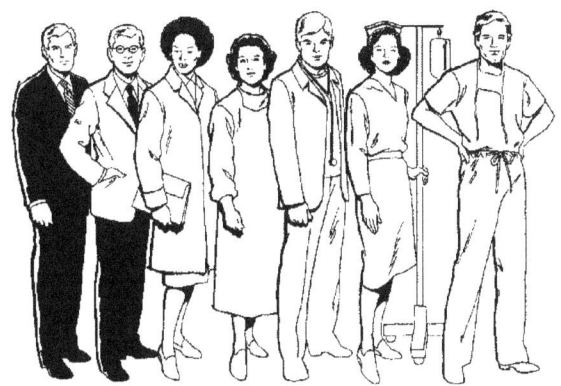

The area of communication exists within all facets of an individual's life; however, the area specific to the medical community and the interactions between physician/dentist and staff is an area that this guide will address. Ineffective communication between the physician/dentist and medical staff can impact the overall efficiency of the medical environment thus affecting multiple areas related to the operation of medical facilities. Some areas related to the human resource department, legal ramifications, and interpersonal skills will be investigated. Attention will be made to the manner in which the patient, staff and physician relationship results in the overall communication process. It is suspected that the level of communication perceived by all is actually not being interpreted by all involved.

Contextual Background: The Emotional Connection

Interactions within the workplace can trigger a variety of emotions that can become apparent when the dynamics of personality and individualism clash. These feelings can then continue to fester until the interaction between all involved becomes convoluted with feelings of hostility. However, a less noticeable or silent incident that may be occurring may actually be related to the inability for a person to communicate their feelings appropriately. As a result, this individual may remain quiet despite their growing animosity toward an individual with whom they work with on a daily basis. Game (2007) contributes that "anxious-ambivalent individuals aim to decrease the psychological distance between themselves and others so may be sensitised to events that could be perceived as evidence that they are not liked or valued" (p. 2). This could be construed as a defense mechanism that a person invokes in order to survive in a stressful work environment and thus the issues may never be openly discussed. Ultimately, this may be a behavior learned early in life and was adopted in order to survive their childhood. As a result, it may very well be likely that the employee and physician relationship is based on the family values and communication skills derived from their family unit.

Effective Leadership

When most people think about effective leaders, many would probably describe these individuals as having the skill of communication and being able to take control of a situation. These two items actually work together and are reliant on one another in order to achieve effective communication. Effective communication involves many facets that closely rely on the interaction between all involved. The combination of personality types and the perceived manner in which communication between each individual materializes is a dependent variable that affects the overall success or failure of quality communication. For instance, a person who has a habit of speaking loudly and maybe even quickly when talking to people could possibly be perceived as being abrasive. However, the individual themselves may not even realize they are speaking in a manner that is abrasive since it may actually be the manner in which they heard this interaction in their own family dynamics as a child. Zachary and Fischler (2007) offer the following components as requirements for effective communication to occur:

1. Feedback - agile leaders master the art of asking for, giving, receiving, accepting, and applying feedback to enhance performance.
2. Accountability - leverages feedback by driving learning, performance, and behavior.
3. Communication - drives the content, clarity, delivery, and timeliness of key information.
4. Trust - enables people to build and sustain relationships.

(p. 1)

Probably one of the toughest aspects for physicians/dentists is to offer constructive feedback to employees within the office environment. This may partly be due to the lack of time in a given day due to the demand of servicing patients and the hectic office environment. Additionally, the skill of providing appropriate feedback may be tied to the life experiences of the individual receiving it. The act of accepting accountability could be difficult for individuals if they are not able to admit they are in the wrong or responsible for a situation involving others. This skill was also probably learned early in

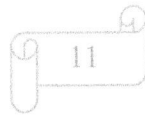

life by interpersonal interaction within social environments. The lack of socialization could actually be a contributing factor as well. The concept of trust may be one of the most difficult since it is usually based on the experience with others. A type of work environment that helps in building trust is an employee-centeredness approach to management. According to Tucker, McCarthy and Benton (2002) "employee-centeredness means that leaders engage in behaviors aimed at building trust, support, and respect among employees, while at the same time working to meet individual employee needs" (p. 225). Depending on the interactions with others in both family and work the task of trust has been developed. The ability to communicate has probably been learned through personal experiences and family interactions as one is raised by their family, as well as been influenced by society. The concept of trust would also be difficult for someone if they lack the proper development of the previous three skills of feedback, accountability, and communication. If they had unfortunate experiences with these during their childhood, it is likely that it would influence their overall experiences within all facets of both their personal and professional life interactions.

It is important to take into consideration that depending on the cultural background of the physicians/dentists and staff there may be differences within their family dynamics during childhood. Also, some belief systems that were adopted may have been incorporated into the adult lives of those particular individuals. These differences may present themselves when daily interactions and communications occur while performing their required functions within the organization. These interactions may then present conflict and animosity if one of the individuals involved feel they are being slighted in some manner. These perceptions could be inferred by the employee based on the tone of voice or the lack of praise for doing a good job by the physician or dental professional. According to McShane and Von Glinow (2008) "when performing our jobs or interacting with co-workers, we experience a variety of emotions that shape our longer-term feelings toward the company, our boss, the job itself, and so on" (p. 108). This differentiation of beliefs of how effective communication must occur could then affect the patients within the office by first-hand observations that there is a conflict between the staff and the physicians/dentists themselves. McShane and Von Glinow (2008) state "emotional labor can be challenging for most of us because it is difficult to conceal true emotions and to display the emotions required by the job" (p. 111). Ultimately, the conflict of communication or the employee's display of frustration with the staff could lead to the loss of patients, as well as the credibility of the medical services within the community.

Another contributing factor that may affect communication may actually be related to the type of career chosen by a person. Clarke-Stewart, Perlmutter, and Friedman (1988) commented that "the complexity of a job may affect personality characteristics such as self-esteem, anxiety, responsiveness to change, moral standards, authoritarianism, intellectual quality of leisure pursuits, and degree of alienation" (pp. 503-504). This may indicate that the training a physician or dentist receives during their education process may actually influence their interpersonal relationships with others due to the increased responsibility that may present itself on a daily basis. In turn, this desensitizing process that may occur during the education process may carry over into the work environment due to social constructions by society and the medical administration's expectations for ethical behaviors. Therefore, the fact that a physician or dentist may appear to be communicating a desired task to staff members may actually only be the result of the product of expectations.

Statement of the Problem

The ultimate impact of ineffective communication could impact a health care facility by legalities, or create challenges for the Human Resource Department. The lack of effective communication and customer service skills could increase an organization's risk for medical malpractice cases. In addition, these attributes of legalities become a burden on the health care facility and would become the challenges for the Human Resource Department. According to Youngberg

(1998) "primary care physicians will need to enhance their communicative skills while directing their focus to the delivery of preventive and routine medical care" (p. 426). With the managed care system in place, physicians/dentists are required to perform procedures to prevent future conditions within a limited time. According to Balint and Shelton (2002)," physicians are subjected to a new set of perverse incentives that reward them for limiting care to patients, in contrast to the fee for service medicine of the past that rewarded them for overtreating patients" (p. 338). This entails physicians and dentists re-evaluating the patient/physician relationship by having to specifically describe the procedures to the patients. To research the validity of communication and customer service in today's health care facilities, the researcher's approach will be taken from a risk management perspective, legal and health care perspective, customer service perspective, training perspective, and Human Resource perspective. This will attempt to show an impact on the primary level because of ineffective communication involving physicians/dentists and their support staff. In addition, the impact on a secondary level could be medical malpractice cases and how ineffective communication affects the Human Resource department.

Research Questions

A series of research questions targeting the areas of communication between the staff, physicians and dentists were given as a random sampling of the medical community in Central and South Florida using an anonymous method of delivery. Participating individuals were directed to a website where they were able to evaluate their present perception(s) of communication within their work environment related to effective communication between patients, staff, physicians and dentists. Additionally, specific areas of focus related to training received by physicians during medical school and the training of staff members was surveyed. The key questions, using a Likert rating system of 1 through 5, were discovered to reflect relevance as outlined below.

Physician/Dentist Key Questions (See Appendix B)

- How would you rate your college medical curriculum in preparing you to communicate with patients?

- How would you rate your college medical curriculum in preparing you to communicate with other healthcare professionals?

Staff Key Questions (See Appendix B)

- How would you rate your written communication skills with health care professionals?
- How would you rate continuing education courses focusing on effective communication with patients?

Significance of Study

The area of communication is an important component within the medical community since the lack of proper communication between the physician/dentist, staff and patients can lead to serious consequences. If a patient is unable to have a conversation with a physician/dentist and understand the treatment plan being prescribed, the patient's condition may worsen and therefore increase the chances for malpractice even though the treatment plan prescribed was valid. Furthermore, if there is miscommunication here, the patient may take steps that are not preventative in nature with the treatment plan, but the patient may accidentally take the wrong amount of medication or at the wrong times, and/or suffer key complications as a result.

On the other hand, if a staff member is unable to interact appropriately with the physician or patient, the treatment plan could become compromised due to the lack of proper documentation or misunderstanding of what was being asked to be done by the physician or dentist. Thus, this lack of communication might unintentionally cause harm to the patient. While this may not have been the intention of the prescribing physician or dentist, they are ultimately responsible for the overall well being of the patient and their treatment regimen.

The ability of effective communication to be conducted within any environment has its place since the lack of proper communication can lead to injury, excess costs related to injury or even death in some instances. Therefore, it is important to incorporate strategies to induce ineffective communication within the business environment. However, the research conducted within this guide focuses primarily on communication within the medical environment between staff, and the physician/dentist.

Research Design and Methodology

It was determined and suspected that there is a breakdown in the communication between physician/dentist, staff and patient when treatment is sought. As a result, a combination of a person-to-person survey and a web-based survey were created to interview the participants in relation to their interactions with physicians and staff members. Since the primary purpose of this study was to measure the level of communication between the physician/dentist and staff members, it was decided by the researcher that patients were not to be included. Instead, a series of questions were designed for physicians and staff that asked similar questions, but were tailored to their daily routines and communications experienced by each.

After the acquisition of the collected data, a standard practice of statistical average measurement was used to identify areas that obtained a rating of less than three, which is considered to be average in the design of the survey scoring system. The survey participants were randomly selected through a coordinator with contacts in a hospital environment within the central Florida area. Additionally, a dentist solicited other professionals in the field to participate in the study within the southern region of Florida. This provided a random distribution of the medical community of physicians, dentists and staff members.

Organization of the Study

In chapter two, the review of literature related to communication within the workplace, medical community was explored with the addition of legal cases resulting in punitive, and liability damages related to the treatment of a patient. Chapter three discusses the lack of effective communication within the employees of a medical treatment facility at both the private practice and hospital level. The data confirmed ineffective communication in a number of areas and the lack of proper education among staff. A summary of the findings and research are addressed within chapter four of this guide.

Chapter 2

Review of Literature

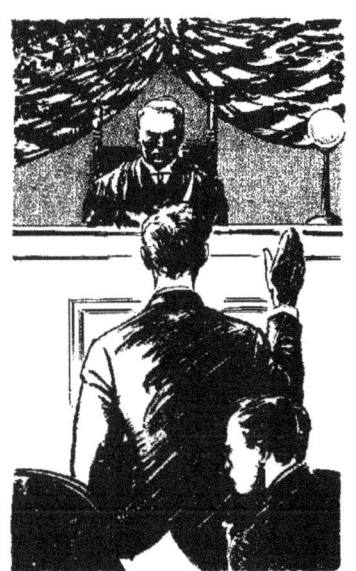

A review of literature was undertaken to validate the impact of health care professionals and the communication process within an organization. There were some interesting aspects that need to be considered, as well as some concepts related to effective communications, that were needed in order to address any deficiencies that might be present within an organizational setting. In order to consider the effectiveness of communication between physicians/dentists and staff, it is also important to reflect on the physician's ability to effectively communicate with patients. Zimmermann and Piccolo (2007) state "one of the crucial challenges of physicians is to be able to grasp and respond to the patients' expressions of emotions, worries, needs and other topics of perceived and immediate importance for the patient" (p. 438). Just as there may be a lack of ability for effective physician/dentist communication to take place between the staff it may also pose as an additional problem related to patients. It is assumed that the effective communication may actually be related to the level of stress occurring in an office on a given day. This would also include tonal fluctuations, sharp responses or derogatory responses to staff member questions and interactions. Congruently, these same behaviors may present themselves when speaking and interacting with patients. These interactions could also impact the overall experience of the patient when considering treatment.

Another point to be considered is the patient's reaction when hearing less than professional reactions directed toward the staff. Conflict in the communication process could impact the patient's relationship with the physician. According to McShane and Von Glinow (2008), "conflict often occurs due to the lack of opportunity, ability, or motivation to communicate effectively" (p. 377). For instance, the patient who is sitting in the waiting room, or in an office waiting for the physician, and over hears the physician/dentist using sharp tones of voice with a staff member could actually negatively impact the patient's point of view of the medical professional providing treatment. Preziosi mentions (2006) "destructive, accusatory feedback only destroys trust and creates hostility" (p. 80). This type of feedback impacts the health care staff and patients observing the behaviors.

Therefore, the impact of communication may actually be perceived or experienced by the patient and have a negative impact on the views of competency and their desire to return for treatment. Additionally, the staff member's perception of the interaction between the physician/dentist and themselves may also lead to depreciated service due to lack of concentration on routine tasks in the office related to communication friction. A customer views their decisions to form a relationship with a company based on their experiences. According to Johnson and Weinstein (2004) "these service encounters affect customer decisions to form long-term relationships with organizations" (p. 5).

The question of whether levels of education between staff and the physician has any bearing on the communication between office personnel is another issue to be considered. Since there is a distinct difference in the amount of education for physicians, dentists and other healthcare professionals it may be possible that the expectations of communication and understanding may actually be vital when communicating treatment recommendations.

Characteristics of Communication

Before addressing the elements needed to foster a functional medical office model for effective communication, the need for an understanding of what communication is will need to be explored. According to Tucker, McCarthy and Benton (2003) "communication is the process of transferring information and understanding from one or more persons to one or more persons" (p. 102). The communication process seems rather simple; however, the manner in which it is accomplished can vary from one individual to another. Additionally, the perceived message that is being communicated can often rely on both objective and subjective systems of understanding. Tucker et. al. (2003) further discusses that "perceptions are the way in which we interpret circumstances—either in an accurate or in a distorted manner" (p. 103). The process of interpretation can be very complex based on a variety of factors, such as, education level, personal belief systems and environmental influences. The combination of these aspects can have an effect on the overall understanding of information being disseminated. These attributes could be reflective of elements related to distorted views, stereotypical viewpoints, and the process of filtering of views. Distorted views can be impacted by the environmental influence exposure either during childhood to adulthood or events occurring during the time of communication, such as, external conversation, equipment noise, or other probable occurrences of distraction. These forms of distractions could inhibit the listener's ability to correctly understand the intended communication between a medical professional and staff member.

Another possible communication breakdown might be based on the variance of educational levels of the physician, staff member, or patient. For instance, if a physician utilizes complex descriptions for patient treatment and the staff member or patient does not fully comprehend the treatment plan due to improper understanding of the instructions given, but are afraid to tell the physician they do not fully understand, the patient may not be given the appropriate treatment, which could lead to further difficulties. Munson (2004) states "patients, being people, do not like to appear stupid and say they don't understand an explanation." (p.11). If the patient does not ask for an explanation, he or she may agree to treatment without understanding the consequences or reasons for the procedure.

Similarly, it may be possible that the physician/dentist has a preconceived stereotypical view of the staff that they are unable to comprehend technical descriptions. Therefore, the physician/dentist resorts to lower–level discussions, which could unknowingly offend the staff members. Another possibility may be related to selective listening skills that actually utilize understanding based on the belief of what is important. The danger with this process is that an important detail could be lost within the translation that could add to a potential conflict later between the physician, dentist, staff member and possibly the patient. These factors could be related to the development of the patient and physician/dentist relationship. According to Balint and Shelton (2002), this could be categorized into six factors:

1. The "basic fault" present in some form in all human beings.

2. The physician's "apostolic function".

3. The "mutual investment company".

4. The role of the physician as a therapeutic agent – the drug "doctor".

5. The "deeper diagnosis".

6. The "conspiracy of anonymity".

(p.340)

The patient's interaction to the social environment and how the physician responds to the reaction of a patient is important in the development of the relationship. Patients react to illnesses differently, some withdraw or some become irate. How the physician reacts to the patient is determined by his or her basic fault. For example, if a patient is very reactive to treatment or an illness, the response from the physician can determine the outcome of the relationship. Balint and Shelton (2002) state "it is also clearly important, therefore, for physicians to try and learn enough about their patients as persons so as to manage their care with due regard for their underlying personalities" (p. 340).

The physician's "apostolic function" relates to the conscious or unconscious influence on the desired outcome that they want the patient to respond. There is an importance of self-awareness that the physician utilizes to ensure his/her behavior is properly received in order to be certain the patient understands the treatment modalities. According to Balint and Shelton (2002), "properly controlled, the apostolic function becomes a mean of patient education and allows opportunities for the patient to educate the physician about his or her person, family, work and other relevant details, and to set forth the patient's own limitations in respect to accommodation to the physician's wishes" (p. 341).

The "mutual investment company" involves the development of the trusting relationship. The physician must be careful to not delve into patient's inter-personal experiences that do not pertain to treatment, because this could impact the therapeutic relationship. This development process helps the role of the physician as a therapeutic agent in determining the right dosage for treatment. Also, it helps with the "deeper diagnosis". In order for a physician to understand the patient's environment to help with the diagnosis, physicians could gain this knowledge through the visits and development of the relationship. Balint and Shelton (2002) communicate "therefore, more effort is needed to learn about each patient's family, home, work place, and so forth so that this deeper diagnosis, which more fully describes the person who has the illness or disease, can be ascertained" (p. 342). This development strengthens the patient/physician relationship. With many physicians being involved with a patient, "conspiracy of anonymity" can occur. This occurs when no one assumes responsibility for a patient's care. This can be a frustrating experience for a patient.

In addition, the form of communication that is involved within the office environment can easily be identified as impacting organizational communication. Tucker, McCarthy, and Benton (2003) defines organizational communication as "any communication that takes place with a total organization—usually formal and written messages, as opposed to informal, interpersonal communication" (p. 108). Organizational communication in today's office environment involves a variety of written and oral communication multiple times a day. Therefore, the fact that miscommunication could occur frequently is apparent. As a result, the need for effective communication needs to be present within any work environment to assist in offsetting the negative impact that could result. Weiss (2001) offers the following for fostering two-way-communication:

- Information disseminated by management must be timely, clear, and useful.

- The significance of data is not always self-evident, nor are management's priorities.

- Participation in a communication system is not a given: people need to be invited to participate, encouraged to speak up, and made to feel valued.

- Good presenters are not born; coaching and practice make a difference.

- Two-way communication is the lifeblood of a communication system; without it, the system becomes malnourished and frail.

(p. 163)

Two-way communication within an organization involves many facets, but the key elements that are presented above are related to proper training and participation by those involved. Therefore, emphasis should be placed on fostering communication and continuous training within the work environment.

Patient Rights to Informed Consent

Another form of communication is related to patient consent for treatment. Fremgen (2009) defines consent as "the voluntary agreement that a patient gives to allow a medically trained person the permission to touch, examine, and perform a treatment" (p. 107). In order for the patient to fully understand the events during an examination, there needs to be a form of proper communication present. As a result, the patient can agree to treatment by giving informed consent for treatment which Fremgen (2009) defines as "the patient agrees to the proposed course or treatment after having been told about the possible consequences of having or not having certain procedures and treatments" (p. 107). However, it is important to point out that if a physician or staff member is unable to effectively communicate the risk of having or not having a particular procedure done and the patient makes a poor judgment as a result, the patient could feel that the tending physician or medical personnel neglected their duties and seek to resolve the situation through monetary gains.

In the case of <u>Johnson v. Kokemoor</u>, involving failure of proper informed consent, it was determined as follows:

A patient cannot make an informed, intelligent decision to consent to a physician's suggested treatment unless the physician discloses what is material to the patient's decision, i.e., all of the viable alternatives and risks of the treatment proposed . . . . In this case information regarding a physician's experience in performing a particular procedure, a physician's risks statistics as compared with those of other physicians who perform that procedure, and the availability of other centers and physicians better able to perform that procedure would have facilitated the plaintiff's awareness of "all of the viable alternatives" available to her thereby aided her exercise of informed consent. (p. 370)

From the <u>Johnson v. Kokemoor</u> case, it can be surmised that the treatment procedure is not the only duty a physician has to their patient to meet their obligation of informed consent, but also their competency to perform the treatment with proficiency. The level of experience also becomes a question of concern since a physician who is not skilled in a particular surgery, may not be able to effectively perform the procedure as competently as a peer who has a record of successful surgeries involving the proposed treatment. This involves referring a patient to another physician that can better assist and treat the patient. Effective communication is important when explaining to the patient the reason they are being referred to another physician. The patient/physician relationship is based on the factor that the physician will provide alternatives for the patient to best meet their needs.

Another interesting aspect related to hospital staff and the liability of the hospital for mistakes was limited to holding employees liable was the case of Bing v. Thunig which determined that a "hospital's liability must be governed by the same principles of law as apply to all other employers" (p. 415). This case determined that since a hospital of modern day now employs staff on a regular basis and not as independent contractors, that they should be held to the same standard as any other business entity in regards to liability. Furrow, Greany, Johnson, Jost and Schwartz (2004) mention "a physician who has staff privileges at a hospital also agrees to abide by hospital bylaws and policies and has therefore agreed to a doctor-patient relationship with whomever comes into the hospital, according to most courts that have considered the issue" (p. 305). This is important because a physician/patient communication can be misconstrued when other health care professionals are involved. The theory of respondeat superior describes that a court can hold another physician or a hospital responsible for the negligence of another. Furrow, Greany, Johnson, Jost and Schwartz (2004) state "under respondeat superior, an employee, who is not liable because of his acts, can be held liable for the wrongful acts of his employees which are committed with the scope of employment" (p. 423). This doctrine enables a patient to recover from the negligence of other physicians and health care professionals involved in treatment. In the case of Darling v. Charleston Community Memorial Hospital, a nurse failed to communicate a patient's condition to a physician. The patient was experiencing numbness in his toes after his knee was set in a cast. He brought this to the attention of a nurse, but she did not communicate this concern to the physician. This resulted in his toes being swollen, numbness, and eventually gangrene to set in because of the nurse's lack of action in contacting the physician about the patient's condition. The patient sued the physician and hospital for negligence due to this incident, which lead to the amputation of the patient's right leg. The court found the nurse, physician, and hospital liable for failure to act. These cases infer the importance of effective communication within a health care facility. The importance of providing patient care within the scope of his/her practice is a key principle to which a physician should adhere. If a physician feels a procedure is outside the scope of practice, a patient should be referred to another physician. Since a physician/patient relationship was developed, the physician has the obligation to communicate to the patient the reasons they are being referred to another health care professional. If the physician or health care staff do not listen to the patient's concerns or provide treatment alternatives, the result can lead to a potential lawsuit.

Failure to Communicate Effectively

The ability to communicate effectively is an important aspect in order to avoid incurring consequences for poor communication practices between the physician and staff. If a patient feels they are the victim of improper treatment or did not fully understand the ramification of a treatment or surgery due to failure of the physician/staff to properly explain the risks, they could choose legal action against the attending physician. Ultimately, the physician/dentist will be held accountable since it is the responsibility for the physician to monitor the behaviors of their staff. Youngberg (1998) offers some guidelines for physicians to follow in regards to the proper development of the patient and physician relationship.

1. Develop the interpersonal interaction by encouraging the antepartum patient to bring a significant other to office visits.

2. Be prepared to spend more time than usual with the patient, especially with primigravidas (first pregnancy).

3. Allow the patient to bring one or two significant others to see the ultrasound viewing, especially if it is done in the physician's office.

4. Always share with the patient the laboratory findings and ultrasound findings regardless of the outcomes.

(p. 290)

These suggested methods are primarily for patients who are experiencing pregnancy, but the information is also applicable for any profession in regards to allowing significant others to participate in the office visit and examination. Additionally, sharing information with others present can actually benefit the physician or dentist since there will be more than one person to recall the information suggested for treatment or diagnosis during the visit. This may be especially true for elderly patients since they may be suffering from hearing or memory issues.

Youngberg (1998) further offers some techniques for making complex information more easily digestible by the client having physicians:

- Pay attention to how much the patient knows and relates any new information to what is already known.

- Use simple, nontechnical language.

- Pictures and charts are useful in explaining anatomy, physiology, pregnancy, and neonatal outcomes.

(p. 290)

These suggestions are useful since it is easy for a physician to forget to explain things in laymen's terms, so a typical patient can easily understand what the physician/dentist is communicating. Patients often do not possess the same level of education, vocabulary or understanding that a medical professional possesses and therefore may have difficulty understanding the suggested treatment being explained to them.

Chapter 3

Overview of the Physician Survey – Medical Curriculum

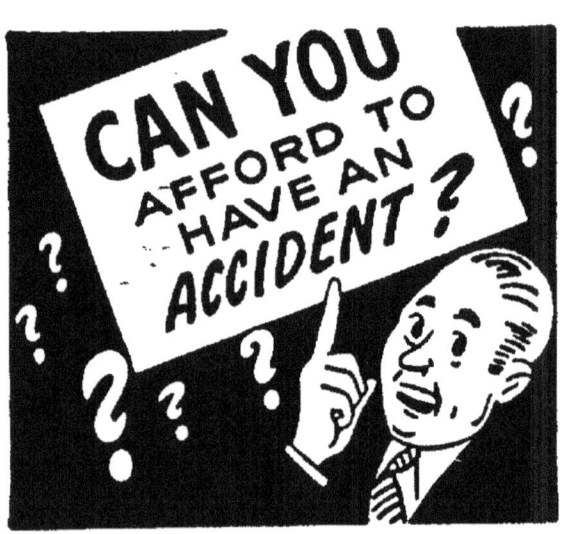

By reviewing the physician survey, the results showed below average scores regarding effective communication. The results showed an average of a 1.33 on a 5.0 scale (Appendix A). Through telephone conversations, and through the survey responses with several physicians and dentists, it was discovered that the college-level medical curriculum involving communication skills were not incorporated into their college course syllabi. In fact, one dentist explained that he learned effective communication in his continuing education courses and effective communication was not included in his medical training (Dentist #1, 2008). This could explain why physicians and dentists have a difficult time trying to relay medical information to their patients. They know the technicalities of their field, but are not confident in how to disseminate the information to their patients.

In addition, another dentist interviewed explained that he had no courses to prepare him on how to open an independent practice. One can infer that if a physician or dentist lacks the ability to set up an independent practice where potentially procedures and policies may be lacking, this could result in ineffective communication skills among the staff members. Lack of business management practices could have a detrimental impact on the patient and the staff. For example, if a patient is using a type of insurance for treatment and the paperwork is not processed efficiently, due to the sole practitioner's inability to manage paperwork, the patient may not be able to have his/her treatment completed in a timely fashion. This could in return lead to future health care issues.

The physician survey demonstrated that physicians and dentists are not prepared to communicate with health care professionals from the education they received during their medical training. The results showed an average of a 2.0 on a 5.0 scale (Appendix A). These results displayed a below average level of effective communication with health care professionals once they leave a college setting. One could deduce that there is potential for a huge impact resulting in a communication barrier between physicians and the health care professionals.

Impact of Communication

From the surveys and telephone conversations with physicians and dentists, the average score was a 3.0 on a scale of 5.0 in how they rated themselves in handling patients who did not understand what they were trying to communicate to them. This could be a concern if a health care professional does not seem comfortable in communicating with patients who do not understand their method of treatment plans. Patients could be consenting to procedures without understanding the complications or impact of a procedure. In addition, the surveys and telephone conversations, showed the average score of a 3.3 on a scale of 5.0 in how they rated themselves in handling health care professionals who did not understand what they were saying (Appendix A). One could conjecture that a health care professional may not feel comfortable in asking for clarification from a physician or dentist when needing a solution to a procedure or policy regarding a patient's health care. The staff member may be apprehensive to communicate concerns if he/she interprets the physician or dentist as not listening to or valuing their input. This could ultimately impact the health care professional and eventually impact the communication of treatment for the patient.

Summary

From the survey and telephone responses, the physicians and dentists rated themselves a 4.0 out of 5.0 as to how communication impacts the patient's visit. There appears to be a conflict between knowing that there is an impact on a patient's visit and the lack of insight into how taking the time to communicate effectively with staff and patients could improve the patient's visit and treatment plans. By spending the extra time to ensure that effective communication is being demonstrated, it would afford a better environment for the patient and health care professional. The details related to the findings will be reviewed related to the level of communication and the impact of deficient use of proper communication in the workplace.

Overview of the Staff Survey

From the participating staff members interviewed, the results indicated that they felt average in their written communication skills with patients. This was based on the scale of a 3.0 on a scale of a 5.0 (Appendix A). From the health care professionals interviewed by telephone, they indicated that they use written communication to break down the patient's invoice and to relay a treatment plan according to the physician's or dentist's directive. This appeared to be helpful in the patient's understanding of their treatment plans and billing information. This type of effective communication could help in reiterating the procedures that will be implemented in the patient's health care plan. In addition, the staff members felt that they were above average in communicating verbally with other health care professionals. This was based on the scale of a 4.0 on a scale of a 5.0 (Appendix A). This could surmise that they felt they were communicating concerns when a patient's treatment was involved. It is interesting to note that physicians viewed themselves higher in communicating with health care professionals instead of written communication with patients.

Most of the health care professionals questioned by telephone were trained in effective communication with patients and other health care professionals by on-the-job training performed by a physician, dentist, co-worker or supervisor. However, it is interesting to note that even though the health care professionals were trained by another health care professional, they rated themselves quite high in trying to explain information to a patient who is not grasping the information. The results showed a 4.67 out of a 5.0 scale. Some of the examples shared were how important it is as health care professionals that they take the time to break technical information down so the patient can understand the medical terms.

One health care professional explained how the dentist speaks so quickly and technical in his communication with his patients that the patients are afraid to ask questions (Participant #1, 2008). By using common language, the staff member helped the patients feel more comfortable. Also, the same staff member mentioned that if a patient does not feel they are heard or does not understand procedures, they are not likely to return to a facility. This healthcare professional personally feels it is their obligation to help the patient understand their treatment plans.

Of the health care professionals surveyed, the results showed the impact of communication on a patient's visit (participant #2, 2008). The surveys showed a 4.33 out of 5.0 scale of how important communication is to a patient's health care experience (Appendix A). There also appeared to be a proactive effort for health care professionals to take responsibility for explaining treatment plans to the patients. Also, one can infer, they feel accountable for ensuring a patient understands the procedures and directives, if the patient does not understand the information portrayed by the physician or dentist.

Recommendations to Improve Communication

From the research and survey results, there appears to be inefficiency in the medical curriculum involving courses in how to communicate with staff and patients. By adding effective communication courses specifically throughout each year of medical school, the physician/dentist would be exposed to how to communicate, how to listen, and how to interpret/analyze the impact of effective communication on the patient's health care. In addition, incorporation into the course curriculum as to how to set up an independent practice, how to set up policies and procedures, and how to channel communication from the physician/dentist through the management team would be a proactive step toward the training of professionals. These courses would also focus on how information would be disseminated to the health care professionals throughout the facility. By streamlining a communication process, this could ensure that employees have a plan of action if they need guidance in a patient's treatment plan. Since, changing a college's curriculum is a timely process due to accreditation processes, the Human Resource department of a facility would need to become involved in implementation of effective communication.

Most employees can often become frustrated when trying to communicate within an organizational setting. According to Preziosi (2006) "without an understanding of some basic communication competence and a support system to communicate effectively and efficiently, employees will frequently feel overwhelmed trying to communicate within the organization" (p. 182). By improving communication, the health care professionals would be able to discuss patient's procedures more openly amongst themselves. By developing educational trainings through the Human Resource department, communication can be improved. In identifying communication styles, it is important to communicate to individuals according to their learning styles. As a physician/dentist, it is important for them to realize that employees have different learning styles. This is useful in trying to explain a procedure, treatment plan or process so the health care professional understands the information being expressed. Preziosi states (2007) "in the neurolinguistic programming model of communication, people are said to process information in three different modes:

visual, auditory and kinesthetic" (p. 42). By recognizing these styles, there is less frustration from the physician/dentist in having a staff member understand what he/she is trying to communicate.

Another area of incorporating open communication is the ability to treat employees as being equals. Health care professionals, as with any employee, want to feel valued for their input. Preziosi emphasizes (2007) "an effective leader speaks to other people as if they were his or her peers" (p. 43). By validating an employee's input and treating them as an equal, the employees would probably take the initiative to add suggestions to improve the health care facility if an issue occurs. Also, by speaking clearly and precisely, it helps to lessen ambiguity. In addition, asking for feedback ensures that the employees' feedback is appreciated. Preziosi mentions (2007) "it often helps to ask the other person if he or she has any comments or questions" (p. 44). This is essential to enabling the health care professionals to express what they do not understand and to be able to add suggestions. The key to effective communication is for a leader to utilize effective feedback when communicating with employees. According to Preziosi (2007) there are several important steps: They consider the other person's perspective.

1. They provide specific, descriptive feedback that can be acted on.
2. They provide descriptive, rather than evaluative, feedback.
3. They do not distort the feedback.
4. They record the feedback when appropriate.
5. They are clear about why they are giving the feedback.
6. They provide the feedback at the appropriate time-usually as soon as possible following the communication or behavior to which the feedback is a response.

(pp. 44-45)

By utilizing these steps, the communication between health care professionals and the physicians/dentists could be improved with appropriate feedback. Also, a supportive type of communication could be promoted by utilizing feedback within the health care facility. This type of approach encompasses the idea that there are various viewpoints in analyzing a solution to an issue. A physician/dentist should embrace the viewpoints of other health care professionals. Preziosi explains (2007) "they understand that both people's perspectives are important in the communication and they encourage honest expression of ideas" (p. 47). By encouraging feedback, the open communication would flourish within the work environment.

Chapter 4

The Results

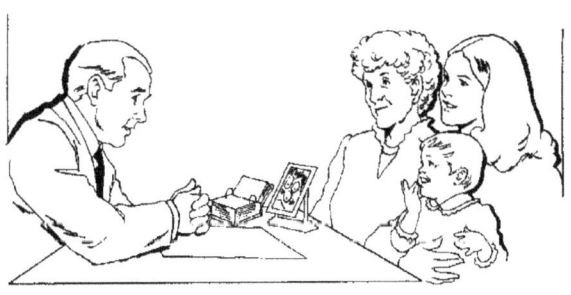

The purpose of this study was to determine whether or not there has been a deficiency in the communication processes between the physician, staff members and patients. The need for strong communication exists between the physician and their staff members in order to facilitate a professional environment and foster a level of confidence within the patient. Additionally, the need for effective communication is important as a protective measure to avoid unwanted confusion related to treatment plans or malpractice lawsuits. This one simple measure can be taken to avoid unnecessary misunderstandings.

Findings

The research conducted appears to support the assumption that there is a deficit between the physicians, dentists and staff members in relationship to the communication process. Additionally, the views of physicians/dentists related to their ability to effectively communicate with staff and a patient may vary from that of the staff, dependent on various factors in the workplace and the individuals' education and training. In many cases, the staff often feels the need to follow-up with patients to ensure their understanding of the proposed treatment, due to the physician's use of technical and medical terminology when explaining the patient's condition or treatment. This sense of responsibility by the staff is probably one reason why there is a lower incidence of treatment confusion for patients, based on reports by the participating staff of this survey. However, it is also important to point out that it may be possible that in other medical settings that staff members may not feel comfortable asking for clarification or taking measure on their own to communicate clearer information to the patient since they may not feel an open communication between the physician and themselves.

Summary

Based on the findings of the research, it appears there is a need to create a manner in which physicians can learn how to effectively communicate with others since physicians surveyed communicated that their curriculum did not properly address the issues related to communication while pursuing their education. One method might be to incorporate a mandatory training provided by an authorized Human Resource company at the state level in order to obtain a medical license for practitioners. This would provide a method of regulation that would help ensure that the physician or dentist is competent when working with patients and staff members. Additionally, the staff should also be exposed to proper communication techniques at state workshops that are required in order to effectively communicate within a medical environment.

The simplest methodology for delivery would be to add effective communication coursework within the physician/dentist medical training program and during the staff education process. However, the inclusion of the curriculum change would take some time to be effectively implemented within the educational system. Therefore, the creation of a secondary training program at the state level might be easier to implement, since it can be changed during licensure process. Additionally, it could be implemented as a continuing education component for those who are already practicing physicians and dentists.

Conclusions

The ability for communication is a necessary component that needs to occur within the medical realms since the research shows a deficient method of communication. By the physician or dentist being able to effectively communicate with patients and staff it can help eliminate the need for follow-up in order to clarify a directive given by the attending physician. This would also help alleviate the potential for error to occur within the translation from staff to patient.

Since the area of medicine is continually under scrutiny, it is important that all methods to boost effective communication be explored. This can be accomplished in a variety of methods such as college curriculum, state-continuing trainings, consulting companies and through the use of an existing Human

Resource department. While these changes would more than likely take time to be successfully implemented, it is important to recognize that the need does exist. Until that time, it is up to the physician/dentist and staff to recognize the need and seek the needed training on their own. Until the importance of the need for effective communication is recognized, it will be necessary for each individual to be responsible for their deficiencies and seek a solution to rectify the process within the health care environment.

10 Key Points to Effective Communication

1. To ensure effective communication is occurring examples, visual aids, etc. should be utilized to reiterate the information being presented.

2. Ask if the patient or health care professional has any questions after information is presented. This enables the individual to ask for clarification.

3. Encourage feedback and suggestions from health care professionals and patients. Being valued as an individual is essential for continuous communication.

4. Be honest with patients. For example, if there are various treatment modalities, inform the patient of the risks and benefits of all the modalities. Patients value honesty.

5. Be cognizant of the interaction of all health care professionals when a patient is in a waiting room or receiving treatment. Patients have time to observe the communication and dynamics of the health care facility or office when determining if they will continue with treatments.

6. Take the time to train new employees in the importance of effective communication. By instilling the importance of a patient centered environment, employees will realize what your expectations are.

7. Provide retraining every four months to ensure employees are in alignment of the communication process. Also, encourage feedback on what may need improving.
8. Establish a process for employees to relay information regarding a patient complaint or potential issue that could occur. For example, a documentation method which can be followed up by a supervisor or yourself.
9. Realize patients and health care professionals learn information differently. Some individuals are visual, others are auditory and others are tactile learners.
10. Be open to new ideas to enhance the communication process. This can be achieved through reading Human Resource articles, seminars on communication or being creative in disseminating communication techniques.

References

Balint, J. and Shelton, W. (2002). Understanding the dynamics of the patient-physician relationship: Balancing the fiduciary and stewardship roles of physicians. The American Journal of Psychoanalysis, 62(4).

Clarke-Stewart, A., Perlmutter, M. & Friedman, S. (1988). Lifelong human development. New York, John Wiley & Sons.

Fremgen, B. F. (2009). Medical law and ethics. (3rd ed.). Pearson-Prentice Hall: Upper Saddle River, New Jersey.

Furrow, B., Greany, T., Johnson, S., Jost, T., and Schwartz, R. (2004). Health law: Cases, materials and problems. Thomson-West, 5th.

Game, A. (2007). Perceiving is believing: Negative affective events and relational models in supervisory relationships. Academy of management proceedings, p. 1-6.

Johnson, W. and Weinstein, A. (2004). Superior customer value in the new economy: Concepts and cases. CRC Press, Boca Raton.

McShane, S. and Von Glinow, M. (2008). Organizational behavior: Emerging realities for the workplace revolution. McGraw-Hill, Boston, 4th.

Munson, R. (2004). Intervention and reflection: Basic issues in medical ethics. 7th, Thomson-Wadsworth, Australia.

Preziosi, R. C. (2006). The 2006 Pfeiffer annual human resource management. John Wiley & Son, San Francisco, CA.

Preziosi, R. C. (2007). The leadership zone: A report and suggestions for action. Llumina Press, Coral Springs, FL.

Tucker, M. L., McCarthy, A. M., Benton, D. A. (2003). The human challenge: Managing yourself and others in organizations. (7th ed.). Prentice Hall: Upper Saddle River, New Jersey.

Weiss, J. W. (2001). Organizational behavior and change: Managing diversity, cross-cultural dynamics and ethics. (2nd ed.). South-Western, Australia.

Youngberg, B. J. (1998). The risk manager's desk reference. (2nd ed.). Maryland: Aspen Publishers, Inc.

Zachary, L., Fischler, L. (2007). The fact model. Leadership excellence, 24(12), p. 20.

Appendix A

Chart 1

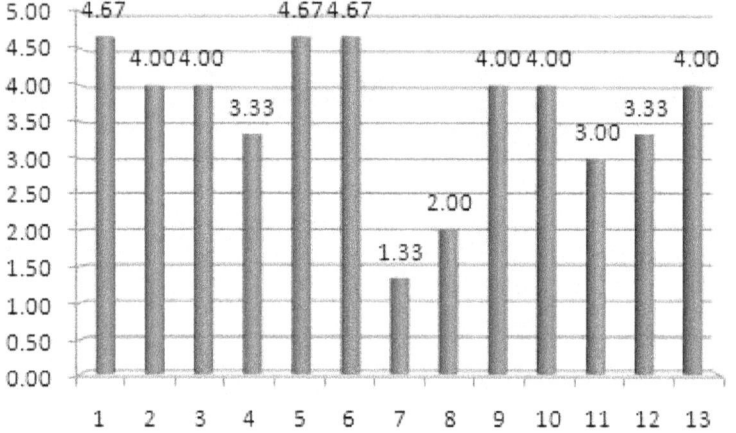

Chart 2

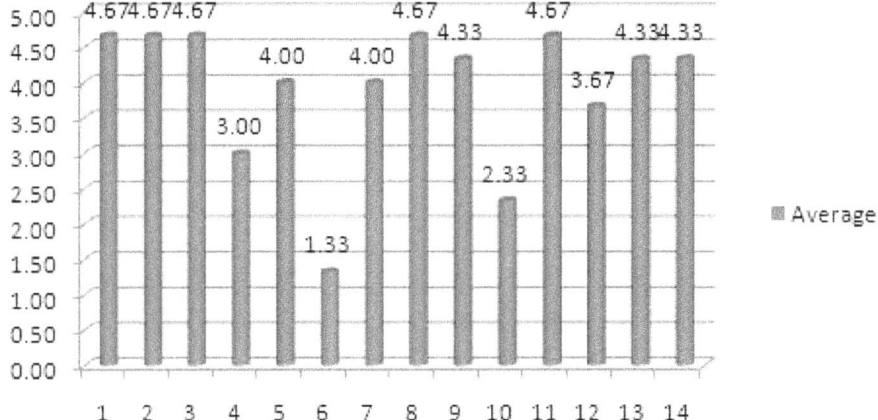

Staff Survey Results

Appendix B

Survey Item 1 - Physician Survey Questions

Physician Survey

Please rate the following questions on a scale **1 – 5**. Also, please fill out the short answer responses as well.

Using the drop boxes below choose the value using the following scale.

5 = excellent   4 = above average   3 = average

2 =below average   1 = poor   0 = not applicable

1. How would you rate yourself as an effective communicator with health care professionals? This includes management, social workers, billing, and other areas.

2. How would you classify yourself as an **effective communicator** with your patients?

3. How would you rate your **verbal communication** skills with your patients?

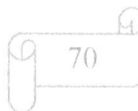

4. How would you rate your **written communication** skills with your patients?

5. How would you rate your **verbal communication** skills with other health care professionals?

6. How would you rate your **written communication** skills with other health care professionals?

7. How would you rate your college medical curriculum in preparing you to communicate with **patients**?

8. How would you rate your college medical curriculum in preparing you to communicate with other **health care professionals**?

9. How would you rate continuing education courses focusing on **effective communication** with other health care professionals?

10. How would you rate continuing education

courses focusing on **effective communication** with patients?

11. How would you rate yourself in handling patients who do not understand what you are communicating to them?

12. How would you rate yourself in handling health care professionals who do not understand what you are communicating to them?

13. How would you rate the communication in the work place impacting the patient's visit?

Please provide short answers for the following questions.

14. Please provide examples of when you have been an effective communicator.

15. Please provide an example of a time when you were faced with a patient who did not understand what you were communicating to them and how you handled that experience.

16. Please provide an example of a time when you were faced with a staff member who did not understand what you were communicating to them and how you handled that experience.

17. How would you rate the impact of miscommunication resulting in a claim against the health care facility?

18. What are some ways you could enhance communication with your staff?

19. What are some ways you could enhance communication with your patients?

20. What do you feel needs to be improved in explaining treatment modalities?

Survey Item 2 – Staff Survey Questions

Staff Survey

Please rate the following questions on a scale 1 – 5. Also, please fill out the short answer responses as well.

Using the drop boxes below choose the value using the following scale.

5 = excellent   4 = above average   3 = average

2 =below average   1 = poor   0 = not applicable

1. How would you rate yourself as an **effective communicator** with other health care professionals? This includes management, social workers, billing, etc.

2. How would you classify yourself as an **effective communicator** with patients?

3. How would you rate your **verbal communication** skills with patients?

4. How would you rate your **written communication**

skills with patients?

5. How would you rate your **verbal communication** skills with health care professionals?

6. How would you rate your **written communication** skills with health care professionals?

7. How would you rate your training in preparing you to communicate with patients?

8. How would you rate your training in preparing you to communicate with other health care professionals?

9. How would you rate continuing education courses focusing on **effective communication** with other health care professionals?

10. How would you rate continuing education courses focusing on **effective communication** with patients?

11. How would you rate yourself in handling patients who do not understand what you are communicating to them?

12. How would you rate yourself in handling health care professionals who do not understand what you are communicating to them?

13. How would you rate the communication in the health care facility in impacting the patient's visit?

14. How would you rate the impact of miscommunication resulting in a claim against the health care facility?

Please provide short answers for the following questions.

15. Please provide an example of a time when you **effectively communicated** with health professionals.

16. Please provide an example of how you communicated with patients who did not understand what was being communicated to them following a

suggested treatment plan by a physician.

17. Please provide an example of how you handled a situation involving a health care professional in which they did not understand what you were communicating to them.

18. What are some ways you could enhance communication with your patients?

www.ingramcontent.com/pod-product-compliance
Lightning Source LLC
Chambersburg PA
CBHW071255170526
45165CB00003B/1353